Defeat Depression

An Independent Program to Quit Feeling like Sh*t.

By

Melanie C. Jenkins

Table of content

Introduction

Everybody encounters bitterness and despondency sooner or later in their lives. Nonetheless, it is more extraordinary and longer-term than regular misery or despondency, which obstructs an individual's capacity to take part in day-to-day exercises. The side effects of sorrow can include loss of interest or delight in beforehand charming exercises, significant changes in craving (either fundamentally decreased or expanded), rest issues (dozing excessively or excessively little), weariness, a sensation of uselessness or sadness, issues with fixation and deciding, and contemplations of self-destruction.

Chapter 1

Definition Of Depression

Depression, in brain science, is a mindset or close-to-home expression that is set apart by sensations of low self-esteem or culpability and a decreased capacity to appreciate life. An individual who is discouraged for the most part encounters a few of the accompanying side effects: sensations of trouble, sadness, or cynicism; brought down confidence and elevated self-deterioration; a reduction or loss of capacity to enjoy standard exercises; decreased energy and imperativeness; gradualness of thought or activity; loss of craving; and upset rest or sleep deprivation. Melancholy contrasts with basic despondency or grieving, which are suitable close-to-home reactions to the deficiency of cherished people or articles. Where there is a clear reason for an individual's misery, discouragement is viewed as present on the off chance that the discouraged state of mind is lopsidedly lengthy or severe. Depression (a significant burdensome problem) is a typical and serious clinical sickness that adversely influences how you feel, how you think, and how you act. Luckily, it is additionally treatable. Despondency causes sensations of misery as well as a deficiency of interest in exercises you once delighted in. It can prompt different profound and actual issues and can diminish your capacity to work at work and at home.

Discouragement influences an expected one out of 15 grown-ups (6.7%) in whatever year. Also, one out of six individuals (16.6%) will encounter misery sooner or later in their life. Depression can happen at whatever point, but generally, first appears during the late youths to mid-20s. Ladies are more probable than men to encounter gloom. A few examinations show that 33% of ladies will encounter a significant burdensome episode in the course of their life. There is a serious level of heritability (roughly 40%) when first-degree family members (guardians/kids/kin) have sadness. Depression Is Not quite the same as Misery or Pain/Loss, The demise of a friend or family member, the cutback of employment, or the cutting off of a friendship are troublesome encounters for an individual to persevere. It is typical for sensations of pity or sorrow to foster because of such circumstances. Those encountering misfortune frequently could depict themselves as being "discouraged." Be that as it may, being miserable isn't equivalent to having misery. The lamenting system is normal and one of a kind to every person and offers a portion of similar elements of misery. Both distress and depression might include extreme bitterness and withdrawal from normal exercises. They are likewise disparate in significant ways:

- In misery, difficult sentiments come in waves, frequently intermixed with positive recollections of the departed. In significant

sorrow, temperament or potential interest
(joy) is diminished for the vast majority of
about fourteen days.

- In misery, confidence is generally kept up.
  In significant sadness, sensations of
  uselessness and self-hatred are normal.

- In misery, contemplations of death might
  surface while considering or fantasizing
  about "joining" the departed cherished one.
In significant depression, contemplations are centered
around taking one's life because of feeling useless or
undeserving of living or being not able to adapt to the
aggravation of despondency. Pain and depression can
coincide For certain individuals, the passing of a friend
or family member, losing employment, or being a
casualty of an actual attack or a significant catastrophe
can prompt sorrow. At the point when anguish and
sadness co-happen, the distress is more serious and
endures longer than misery without sorrow. Recognizing
distress and gloom is significant and can help individuals
in getting the assistance, backing, or treatment they
need.

Risk Elements For Depression

Depression can impact anyone, even a person who appears to live in decently ideal circumstances.
A few elements can assume a part in sadness:

Natural Chemistry: Contrasts in specific synthetic compounds in the mind might add to the side effects of wretchedness.

Hereditary Qualities: Wretchedness can run in families. For instance, in the event that one indistinguishable twin has sorrow, the other has a 70 percent chance of having the sickness at some point throughout everyday life.

Character: Individuals with low confidence, who are effortlessly wrecked by pressure, or who are for the most part critical have all the earmarks of being bound to encounter misery.

Ecological Variables: Ceaseless openness to savagery, disregard, misuse, or neediness might make certain individuals more defenseless against misery. Discouragement represents more handicaps overall than some other condition during the center long stretches of adulthood as a matter of fact, the significant burdensome problem is presently the main source of incapacity overall For some with burdensome episodes, times of misery might determine in half a month or months. In any case, it has been assessed that, for 30 to 50 percent of grown-ups, despondency is repetitive or ongoing if one neglects to determine Unexpectedly, discouragement is maybe perhaps of the most really treated mental problem and, whenever perceived early, it tends to be forestalled.

Chapter 2

Types and Side Effects Of Depression

It's generally expected to feel down now and again, however on the off chance that you're miserable more often than not and it influences your day-to-day existence, you might have clinical gloom. It's a condition you can treat with medication, conversing with a specialist, and changes to your way of life.
There is a wide range of sorts of despondency. Occasions in your day-to-day existence cause some, and synthetic changes in your mind cause others.

A few different side effects you could have are:
- Loss of interest or delight in your exercises
- Weight reduction or gain
- Inconvenience getting to rest or feeling tired during the day
- Feeling anxious and upset, or, in all likelihood extremely languid and dialed back actually or intellectually
- Being drained and without energy
- Feeling useless or remorseful
- Inconvenience thinking or simply deciding
- Considerations of self-destruction.

Significant depression is diversely searched in various individuals. Contingent upon how your downturn causes you to feel, it very well may be;

Despairing: You feel seriously miserable and lose interest in the exercises you used to appreciate. You feel awful in any event when beneficial things occur. You could likewise:

Feel especially down in the mornings
Get in shape
Rest ineffectively
Have self-destructive considerations.

Assuming you have melancholic depression, your side effects may be most obviously terrible in the mornings when you first wake up. Consider having somebody assist you with your most memorable assignments of the day. Make a point to eat consistently regardless of whether you feel hungry.

Restless Trouble: You feel tense and fretful most days. You experience difficulty concentrating because you're concerned that something dreadful could occur, and you feel like you could fail to keep a grip on yourself. Talk therapy can help. You'll meet with an emotional well-being expert who will assist you with tracking down ways of dealing with your downturn.

Tenacious Burdensome Problem: Assuming you have discouragement that goes on for quite some time or longer, it's called a persevering burdensome problem.

This term is utilized to portray two circumstances recently known as dysthymia (poor quality diligent despondency) and ongoing significant sadness.
You might have side effects, for example,

Change in your hunger (not eating enough or gorging)
Dozing excessively or excessively little
Absence of energy, or exhaustion
Low confidence
Inconvenience focusing or deciding
Feeling sad.

Bipolar Turmoil: Somebody with bipolar turmoil, which is additionally at times called "hyper despondency," has temperament episodes that reach from limits of high energy with an "up" state of mind to low "burdensome" periods.
At the point when you're in the low stage, you'll have the side effects of significant depression.
Prescription can assist with managing your emotional episodes. Whether you're in a high or a low period,

Occasional Full Of Feeling Problem:
(occasional gloom): This is a type of significant
burdensome problem that normally emerges throughout
the fall and winter and disappears throughout the spring
and summer.

Pre-birth depression and post-pregnancy: Pre-birth
depression is discouragement that occurs during
pregnancy. Postpartum anxiety is discouragement that
creates within four weeks of conveying a child.

Abnormal depression: Side effects of this condition,
otherwise called significant burdensome issues with
abnormal highlights, shift somewhat from "normal"
misery. The primary distinction is an impermanent state
of mind improvement in light of positive occasions
(temperament reactivity). Other key side effects
incorporate expanded hunger and dismissal
responsiveness.

Chapter 3

What Causes Despondency? (Depression)

There are a few thoughts regarding what causes melancholy. It can change a ton between various individuals, and for certain individuals, a blend of various variables might cause their downturn. Some find that they become discouraged with next to no undeniable explanation.

In this part you can track down data on the accompanying potential reasons for misery:

- Adolescence encounters
- Other psychological well-being issues
- Life-altering situations
- Actual medical conditions
- Hereditary legacy
- Medicine, sporting medications, and liquor
- Rest, diet, and exercise.

Youth Encounters

There is a great proof to demonstrate the way that going through troublesome encounters in your life as a youngster can make you helpless against encountering discouragement further down the road. This could be:

Physical, Sexual, or Psychological Mistreatment

Research demonstrates the way that going through loads of more modest testing encounters can bigger affect your weakness to depression than encountering one significant awful accident.

Troublesome encounters during your experience growing up can hugely affect your confidence and how you figured out how to adapt to troublesome feelings and circumstances. This can cause you to feel less ready to adapt to life's promising and less promising times and lead to depression sometime down the road.

Life Altering Situations

As a rule, you could find your downturn has been set off by an unwanted, unpleasant, or horrible mishap. This could be:

- Losing your employment or joblessness
- The conclusion of a friendship
- Deprivation
- Significant life-altering events, such as evolving position, moving house, or getting hitched
- Being truly or physically attacked
- Being tormented or manhandled, including encountering prejudice.

Negative encounters cause sadness, yet the way that we manage them. If you don't have a lot of help to assist you with adapting to the troublesome feelings that

accompany these occasions, or then again assuming
you're now managing other tough spots, you could find
that a low state of mind forms into depression health
problems.

Chronic weakness can add to your gamble of creating
misery.
Numerous medical conditions can be very challenging to
make due to and can immensely affect your mindset.
These could be:

Actual Medical Conditions
Actual medical conditions essentially change your way
of life. You may be offered help for your psychological
well-being simultaneously as you are treated for an
actual medical condition, as a component of your general
therapy. Some actual medical issues can cause
depression:

- Conditions influencing the mind and sensory
  system
- Hormonal issues, particularly thyroid and
  parathyroid issues
- Side effects connecting with the period or
  the menopause
- Low glucose
- Rest issues.

Hereditary Legacy

Albeit no particular qualities for discouragement have been distinguished, research has shown that on the off chance that you have a nearby relative with depression, you are bound to encounter depression yourself.
While this may be brought about by our science, this connection could likewise be because we normally gain conduct and approaches to adapting from individuals around us as we grow up.

Medicine, Sporting Medications, and Liquor.

Depression can be a result of various medications. If you are feeling discouraged in the wake of beginning any sort of drug, really take a look at the patient data handout to see whether sadness is a secondary effect. On the off chance that you think a medication is causing your downturn, you can converse with your primary care physician about taking another option, particularly on the off chance that you are anticipating that your treatment should endure a little time. Alcohol and sporting medications can both cause discouragement. In spite of the fact that you could at first use them to cheer yourself up, or to divert yourself, they can aggravate you generally speaking.

Rest, Diet, and Exercise

A terrible eating routine and absence of rest and exercise can influence your mindset, and make it harder for you to adapt to troublesome things happening in your life. Albeit a horrible eating routine, or not getting sufficient rest or exercise, can't straightforwardly cause depression, they can make you more helpless against creating it.

Chapter 4

Self-Improvement For Conquering Despondency (Depression)

8 Self-Improvement Solutions to Reduce the Effects of Dejection; It's difficult and crippling to be dejected. Every year, an estimated 10% of adults in the US suffer from the negative side effects of depression, which can lead to arguments within families, decreased productivity at work, and a sense of hopelessness in both the affected person and those around them. While seeking professional clinical help for depression is always a good idea, especially if the disease is severe, there are also many non-clinical measures a person may do on their own to lessen the effects of depression. Several counselors and specialists encourage dejected patients to take steps like these in addition to guidance and treatment.

Here are eight activities that a person who is dejected can engage in:

1. Take Up Some Exercise

Many rational analyses of depression find that exercise is just as effective as medication at reducing mild to moderate dejection. Beyond alleviating depression's negative effects, the technique has other beneficial benefits like improved cardiovascular health, weight loss, and a lower risk of contracting a variety of chronic diseases.

It is best to start small and complete something enjoyable because practicing when dejected is often very tough. Suitable forms of activities for reducing misery include taking daily brief walks, working out for ten minutes at home, and moving to music.

The technique helps with the negative consequences of sorrow because it increases the brain's production of endorphins. Yes, even a few minutes per day of easy exercise.

2. Negative Factors To Consider

People commonly engage in bad thinking when they are discouraged. In a discouraged person's mind, thoughts like "I'm a disappointment," "Nobody likes me," or "I'll always have this impression" are common. These kinds of pessimistic views encourage the feeling of misery by becoming an unconscious inclination.

Testing negative considerations with positive reasoning is a simple arrangement. To test the idea that "I'll continually feel as such," for instance, ask yourself, "How do I have at least some idea of that?" on the other hand review when you have an in any case outlook on presence. We typically accept our thoughts without putting them to the test. Nonetheless, the adage "Don't entirely accept all that you think" has a lot of cunning.

3. Consume a Variety Of Healthy Foods Consistently

When someone gets discouraged, they regularly and almost always eat inefficiently. Sweet, sour, and high-fat unhealthy foods can temporarily make you feel better, but in the long run they raise your blood sugar, make you gain weight, and give you a bad attitude.

The plan is to locate healthy food options you enjoy, make sure there are enough available nearby and consume these options regularly. As long as you don't have a food sensitivity or another negative reaction to the meal, new natural products, mixed greens, lean meats, smooth fish like salmon, and whole grain bread are excellent choices.

Finding healthy eating options you enjoy is the main goal.

4. Get Enough Sleep

Anxiety and sadness both have a role in insomnia, which can involve problems getting to sleep and staying asleep. Making changes in accordance with your routine might assist you with dozing all the more adequately throughout the evening. For instance,

go to bed every night at the same time.

In the bedroom, avoid using a computer or TV.

Before going to bed, wait at least an hour to eat.

Ensure that the bedroom is as silent and dark as you can.

Ensure the room is at an agreeable temperature. For at least two hours before going to bed, abstain from all caffeine-containing beverages.

Our body and cerebrum should snooze requests to restore, mend, and recover. A restful night's sleep each night enhances general health and energy level which reduces the symptoms of depression.

5. Often Sip Water

All significant physical processes require water. Enough water should be consumed each day to help the body eliminate toxins, improve the function of internal organs, and even sharpen judgment.

Many people neglect to drink enough water and then overindulge in sodas, stimulating beverages, and alcoholic beverages. Certain types of drinks cause the body to lose water, which results in dehydration.

Consider the following alternatives if drinking plain water is a test:

enhanced sparkling water,

cutting a lemon, lime, or fresh ginger root and adding it to ice water;

Natural teas include mint, chamomile, ginger, hibiscus, rooibos, or jasmine that are hot or cold. A spoonful or two of natural product juice can be added to water to improve the flavor.

Adults require an additional couple of quarts of fluid per day in addition to what they consume in food for optimal health. Keeping your body strong reduces depressive feelings.

6. Introduce A Change To Routine Practice

When someone is depressed, they typically adopt a standard that promotes the negative impacts of depression. For instance, a dejected person might get up, go to work, come home, watch the same television shows every night, and then binge on unhealthy food before going to bed. Such a schedule may cause someone to continually second-guess their decisions. Introducing routine improvement need not be complicated. For instance, when you get home from work, focus on taking a quick stroll rather than rushing straight to the television. Make a small effort to eat a better feast rather than a terrible dinner.

Dopamine is a key mind chemical linked to feelings of happiness, and altering schedules can help reorganize dopamine pathways in the brain. Routine improvements don't necessarily need to be significant to have an impact.

7. Chuckling

Chuckling is one more strategy for expanding dopamine in the cerebrum. Plunking down and watching satire shows or films, understanding jokes, snickering with others, or just pondering entertaining things that outcome in chuckling can all lift dopamine levels and help with the side effects of depression.

8. Help Another Person

There are areas of strength for when we are discouraged to become egotistical. Our concerns pose a potential threat to us, adding to the sensation of being overpowered. A straightforward arrangement is to benefit someone else or to deal with a pet creature.

Calling a companion to ask how they are doing, chipping in at a nearby foundation, assisting a neighbor with yard work, or embracing a pet are a couple of models. At the point when we help other people, it raises our confidence, and we additionally get our personalities off of our difficulties. Any respite from discouraged sentiments can help with working on sure reasoning and hoisting state of mind. Beginning these self-improvement activities might appear to be trying at first for a discouraged individual. Nonetheless, making even a little change every day can rapidly gather speed and increment energy as side effects of discouragement start to die down. Taking little, everyday strides toward a better life can essentially affect the decrease of gentle to direct side effects of misery.

7 Food Sources You Ought to Keep Away From In the Event that You Have Sadness

You presumably definitely realize that diet tremendously affects your mental and mental state. It's not shocking then that downturn is a psychological well-being problem frequently joined by unfortunate dietary patterns.

Embracing a sound way of life can demonstrate a genuine test when you are battling with significant pity, absence of energy, touchiness, and sleep deprivation. Nonetheless, barring unsafe food varieties from your eating regimen is the most important move toward a better cerebrum and psyche.

Thus, here's a rundown of food sources and drinks you ought to avoid with regard to the menu to limit glucose variances, mindset swings, and serious burdensome side effects.

Liquor

Individuals who battle with low temperament and energy frequently use liquor as a type of self-medicine to encourage them. Notwithstanding, when alcoholic impacts die down, they feel surprisingly more terrible than previously, so an endless loop is made. Liquor fills in as a depressant, meaning it stifles your focal sensory system and obstructs how you process feelings. It additionally influences rest quality, so in the event that you are now dozing ineffectively, avoid liquor utilization however much as could reasonably be expected.

Espresso

Caffeine can influence individuals in various ways. In the event that your body doesn't endure it well, you might encounter apprehension, crabbiness, and an expanded pulse. You ought to eliminate your espresso admission continuously to limit the adverse consequences of caffeine withdrawal. Have a go at supplanting some espresso with different refreshments so as not to feel totally denied. Choose decaf, or, far superior, natural homegrown tea - its normal properties can help your sensory system, work on your mindset, and assist you with dozing better.

Caffeinated Beverages and Soft Drinks

Depression frequently accompanies steady weakness and weariness, so caffeinated drinks frequently show up as a brief arrangement. In any case, they cause more damage than great; the blend of caffeine, sugar, and counterfeit sugars can cause expanded heartbeat and rest disturbances. Standard bubbly beverages can likewise be dangerous, as they have no healthful advantages while containing a reasonable portion of sugar and sugar. Diet soft drinks are no greater for you, and their caffeine content is likewise liable to build uneasiness and leave you feeling considerably more discouraged.

Natural Product Juices

Natural product juice can offer a fast shot in the arm, yet the cost you pay is steep. Your glucose drops quickly, and you are left inclination ravenous and more aggravated than previously. In opposition to prevalent thinking, natural product juices don't extinguish your thirst successfully, so drinking heaps of water is a much better practice. Eating natural entirely organic products is likewise a superior other option; the fiber content keeps you full and balances your glucose as well as your mindset.

Handled Food Sources

Handled food sources are reasonable, effectively available, and profoundly attractive. They require very little or no readiness, so individuals who don't have the inspiration or the energy to plan nutritious, even feasts at home frequently resort to them. By the way, these kinds of food varieties are the encapsulation of all that is off with the cutting-edge Western eating regimen. They are high in added substances, sugar, salt, and calories. Customary utilization increments irritation all through the body, including the cerebrum. Delayed fiery reactions can build the gamble of discouragement and lead to craving changes, weakness, mental hindrance, rest unsettling influences, negative state of mind, and social withdrawal.

Salad Dressings and Ketchup

Premade salad dressings and sauces are loaded with sugar in different structures, for example, fixings like corn syrup. Indeed, even the alleged "sans sugar" items contain aspartame, a fake sugar related to expanded side effects of uneasiness and depression. Ketchup is likewise a terrible decision in light of its outstandingly high sugar content (four grams for every tablespoon). Custom-made natural dressings and salsa are your ideal choice since you set them up without any preparation and control every one of the fixings you put in them.

Trans Fats

Trans fats are found in a wide assortment of normal items like bundled prepared products, handled food sources, margarine, and broiling oil utilized for preparing cheap food. They can hook onto the blood vessel walls and cause atherosclerosis and an expanded gamble of coronary illness. They are likewise connected to a higher gamble of depression, as well as sensations of hostility and crabbiness. It is additionally conceivable that these mixtures decrease serotonin (frequently called "the blissful chemical") creation in the cerebrum. Substitute trans fats with avocado oil to support your cerebrum and work on your mindset.

Way of life changes, including a more nutritious eating regimen, is urgent for misery recuperation and counteraction. Assuming that you are now managing burdensome side effects, low inspiration could keep you from embracing better dietary patterns. By and by, it's memorable and vital that even little changes can have positive long-haul impacts. Try not to entice yet hurtful food sources and beverages whenever the situation allows and you have made the initial step to work on physical.

Chapter 5

Instructions On How To Stay Away From Depression During the Covid Outbreak

The episode of new Covid has impacted numerous areas of day-to-day existence, including psychological wellness. With the unexpected disturbance of our schedules and the new standard of social separation, life as far as we might be concerned has decisively changed surprisingly fast. Unexpectedly, a considerable lot of us are confronting the pressure of the news and its effect on our funds alone, seriously endangering us for depression during the Covid flare-up.

"This is an amazing coincidence for melancholy and anxiety. With everything going on, individuals can wind up ruminating, feeling miserable and powerless, and, at last, discouraged. We are confronting a public injury, whether it's the feeling of dread toward being contaminated or tainting another person or the financial slump, and many individuals are isolated. Those who as of now battle with melancholy and tension might find what is going on worsens their sentiments. Other people who are accustomed to keeping occupied may out of nowhere find themselves alone with their viewpoints more, and missing loved ones beyond their family. While the need to keep social separation makes a few obstructions, there are explicit advances you can take to "make the best of horrible,"

Track Down The Expectation

This might sound inconceivable during a troublesome time, yet rather than think, "This is a mind-blowing reminder," take it step by step or step by step. Make a stride back and see if there is motivation to be confident. For people feeling the monetary effect of the Covid, a silver lining might be particularly elusive during this time. Attempt to change your mentality: In the event that you've lost work, as opposed to considering this to be an extremely durable circumstance, consider it in the middle between getting back to work. When the pandemic crisis is finished, there will be repressed interest. Everybody will be anxious to go out to cafés and travel, so large numbers of those positions will be there in the future.

Keep A Timetable

Bunches of people have lost their typical schedules, and that unstructured time can likewise prompt rumination and latency, high gamble factors for sadness. Plan your day, down to the hour. Toward the day's end, verify things and make a plan for the day the following day, so you can anticipate things. Make a bunch of objectives for the week and for the month, then make some more extended-term objectives.

It's particularly critical to keep structure assuming that you've lost your employment. It's normal for individuals to be disturbed when they're jobless. Notwithstanding the monetary issues, they lose the design in their lives. One approach to adapting is to structure your time.

Be Useful With Your Available Energy
As opposed to considering segregating as being in jail, you can consider it to be having all the more extra energy. Attempt to track down snapshots of bliss in this opportunity. Create a rundown of exercises you can participate in. You can in any case go outside to work out or go online to track down an activity or yoga video. Peruse the books and watch the motion pictures you've been important to. Find time for the errands you've put off, such as cleaning your storage rooms. Become inventive about cooking. Perhaps you've been requesting takeout for some time and failed to remember you have a kitchen.

A gamble that accompanies segregation and detachment is the propensity to ruminate and have considerations like: "For what reason is this event? This is so horrendous, I can't stand it." You can either ruminate or you can issue a settlement. Ask yourself: "What's the issue? I'm exhausted, I'm in confinement. Alright, so I could work out, I can contact individuals, I can make arrangements, and finish errands. I can view this as a test to distinguish present moment and long haul objectives."

Associate With Others (regardless of whether not up close and personal)

Since we are holding up doesn't mean we want to separate ourselves really. Make a rundown of companions, including some you haven't had contact with in quite a while, and utilize your telephone as a phone. Set up a standard time every day to contact individuals, and timetable virtual social gatherings on internet-based stages to talk or perhaps mess around. You could begin a book club online with your companions.

In the event that you have a friend or family member in the medical clinic or going through a difficult time, it's not difficult to feel defenseless, particularly on the off chance that you can't visit or assist them with feeling improved. Yet, you can continuously tell individuals you love them and care about them. We frequently underrate that it is so essential to communicate association, love, and appreciation. Also, we can do that on a continuous premise, not right when somebody is wiped out.

Reexamine Your Point Of View
It's alright to feel upset and to recognize to yourself and to others these are troublesome times. However, this could be a potential chance to ponder what you esteem or truly maintain that should do with your life. On the off chance that you view this period as a deliberate act of not going out to cafés and bars, you might understand you can flourish without those schedules. At the point when the pandemic dies down and the crisis is lifted, you might find you value the opportunity to go to the rec center or spend time with your companions significantly more.

The pandemic might raise contemplations of mortality. A positive perspective about mortality is to perceive what's truly critical to you throughout everyday life, which may be having significant connections, adding to the improvement of society, or being inventive. Since we can't collaborate with individuals up close and personal doesn't mean we should be segregated and uninvolved. It's not unexpected to feel restless, yet we can deal with the experience, keep dynamic and associated, keep up with as a very remarkable everyday practice as possible, and fabricate flexibility as we climate the emergency.

The most effective method to Adapt To Anguish In the midst of Coronavirus.
Realize your sentiments are legitimate. Depression is chaotic and a characteristic reaction to misfortune. There are no set-in-stone ways of encountering it. There are, obviously, shared characteristics, yet our reaction to misfortune is different for each individual and furthermore for every individual we lose. As a rule, despondency starts intensely with extraordinary feelings, engrossing considerations, actual responses, and ways of behaving zeroed in on regarding, really focusing on, and feeling near the deprived. Over the long run, as we adjust to misfortune by embracing its situation and reestablishing our prosperity, melancholy is coordinated and tracks down a spot in our life.

Comprehending That Unexpected misfortune is stunning and challenging to fathom. After a difficult misfortune, it's not difficult to envision ways it didn't need to work out. This is something nearly everybody does. At the point when a friend or family member kicks the bucket unexpectedly, under troublesome conditions, as is occurring with the Coronavirus passing, the propensity to become involved with envisioning a wide range of elective situations is significantly more grounded. This is known as a "derailer" because it can divert a versatile recuperating process.

Utilize The Principles Of The Tranquility Supplication

You really want to acknowledge what you can't change; this implies tolerating the passing yet in addition the presence of the pandemic and its ramifications. You likewise need boldness, imagination, and guts to change your best. This implies tracking down ways of re-establishing your prosperity and adapting to the pandemic, which incorporates three essential parts:
1) acting in manners that are predictable with significant individual qualities or profoundly held interests,
2) feeling capable to face and address significant difficulties throughout everyday life, and
 3) having a feeling of having a place and matter on the planet.

Look out for contemplations that can wreck your recuperating cycle. Assuming they take an excess of room to you, particular sorts of regular considerations, sentiments, or ways of behaving can crash mending during intense lamenting. These incorporate fighting the demise; self-fault, culpability, outrage, or disgrace; envisioning ways things might have gone in an unexpected way; losing confidence in yourself or others; over-the-top evasion of tokens of misfortune; and outrageous social seclusion.

Try not to allow culpability to overpower you. You will probably discover yourself feeling survivor culpability. This is exceptionally normal, however, it is something special to notice and focus on while attempting to not allow it to dominate and direct your decisions as you push ahead. At the end of the day, you really want to permit yourself to have bliss and fulfillment in your life once more. That could take some time. Simply make an effort not to keep yourself away from having positive feelings and enjoying them.

Conclusion

In spite of the fact that there is still a lot of data to be accumulated, obviously, there is a case for the utilization of different hallucinogens as a treatment for gloom, Even as far back as the 1940s, researchers were searching for remedial methodologies for what are currently for the most part unlawful and restricted substances that were exploited for their sporting advantages. Today, those reviews are showing guarantee and what's in store is splendid. With a lot of supporting data and exploration from different solid sources to back up the advantages of this treatment for gloom and PTSD, as well as other psychological wellness conditions. It's inevitable before the others get additional time in the examination spotlight and look for their own way. The mind is as yet a baffling monster, generally, and for all that, we realize there is something else to learn. Nonetheless, we really do realize that injury and state of mind problems can influence the cerebrum's capacity to appropriately deal with feelings or handle things. By utilizing hallucinogens to decrease those obstacles and basically "bring down the walls", individuals will actually want to get to the foundation of their issues and find a goal significantly more rapidly and successfully. This is, obviously, the expectation of the defenders for hallucinogens as a treatment for depression, which offers another universe of desire to the people who presently can't seem to track down alleviation, and for the individuals who realize that their biggest issue is having the option to escape their own specific manner. For the

individuals who need an alternate way, it may not be
some time before we see this as a choice that is
accessible.